GASTRITIS HEALING COOKBOOK 2024

A New Complete Guide to Heal Gastritis and Improve Your Stomach Health

Magdalene Charles

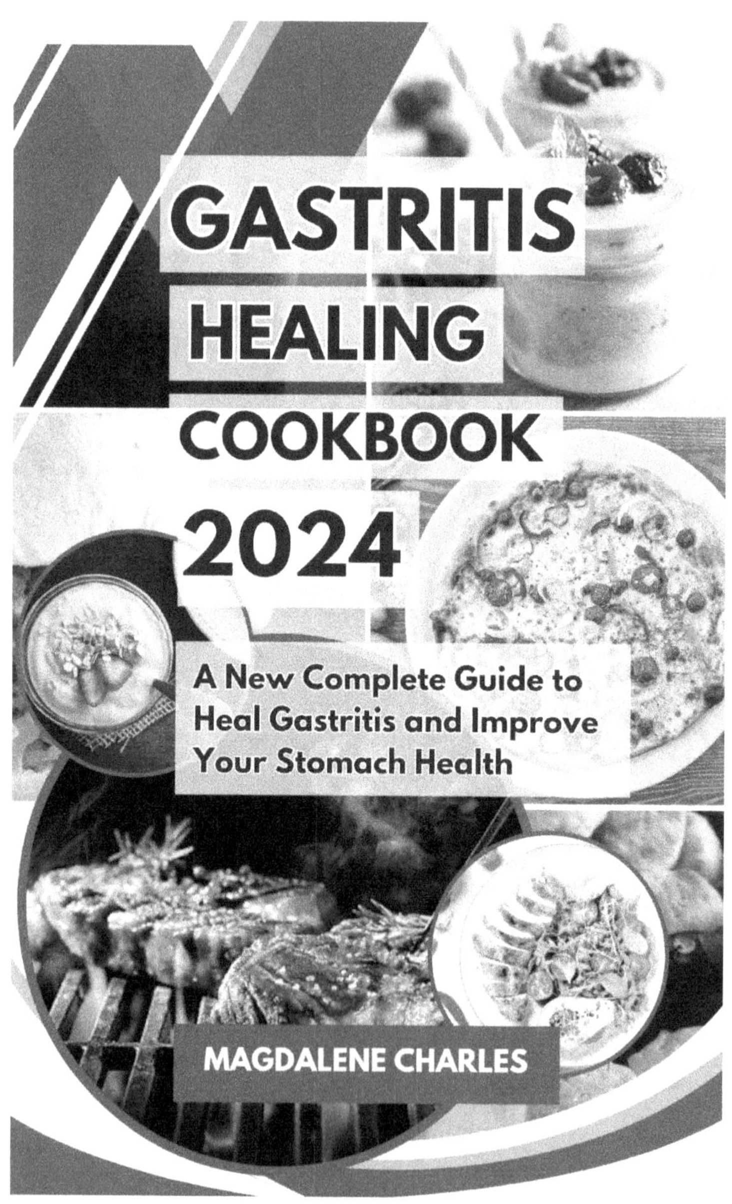

GASTRITIS
HEALING
COOKBOOK
2024
A New Complete Guide to
Heal Gastritis and Improve
Your Stomach Health
MAGDALENE CHARLES

TABLE OF CONTENT

Overview

The term "gastritis" refers to a collection of conditions that all share the inflammation of the stomach mucosa. In fact, today's gastritis not only affects people of all racial, age, and socioeconomic backgrounds, but it also takes many forms. For example, some patients with gastritis complain of simple, transient heartburn; others, on the other hand, experience dyspepsia, aerophagia, and appetite loss, which can progress to severe, incapacitating symptoms like vomiting, meteorism, diarrhea, and abdominal cramps. The kind of symptoms and their frequency are greatly influenced by the triggering factor. Fortunately, changing one's lifestyle can usually promptly cure moderate gastritis.

On the other hand, more harsh therapy may be required in situations where the disease assumes a chronic or particularly aggressive connotation. In both situations, particularly if severe, the malaise felt needs to be brought to the doctor's attention in order to prevent needless suffering and because, in some cases, the onset of heartburn, cramps, or abdominal pain may indicate a more serious ailment that carries serious risks for general health. Let's learn about the various illnesses that may cause it, the most typical signs that might help identify it, potential cures, and the importance of a balanced diet.

CHAPTER 1

WHAT IS GASTRITIS

Gastritis is a condition that can be either acute or chronic and is defined by inflammation of the stomach walls along with other symptoms like bloating, cramping, nausea, and gas. Since gastritis is a complex disorder influenced by a number of factors, it frequently results from more than one cause. Not surprisingly, a hereditary susceptibility combined with an improper diet and lifestyle are frequently the underlying causes of issues. Another etiological element that should be taken into consideration is stress, which is essentially ubiquitous in the Western population today and affects people of all ages and genders equally.

Infections, smoking, a sedentary lifestyle, a lack of food education, climate change, and a fast-paced work environment can all exacerbate gastritis.

Classification and causes

A mucous membrane that serves as a barrier against the acids needed for digestion often covers the walls of the stomach. The digestive juices can harm and inflame the stomach walls, leading to gastritis, since the acids in the stomach are so caustic that, in the absence of sufficient protection, they would end up digesting the stomach itself.
Among the several reasons, we identify:

Helicobacter pylori infection

Gastric ulcers are most commonly caused by Helicobacter pylori infection, which also causes many cases of gastritis, most of which are chronic in nature. This bacterium is thought to have spread from person to person and infected half of the world's population. Though the majority of infected individuals may not experience infection-related consequences, in some cases the bacterium can cause the interior mucosa of the stomach to tear, altering the gastric walls. The reason for the 20% of the population that solely has a Helicobacter pylori infection is unknown. However, medical professionals think that a person's susceptibility to the bacteria may run in the family or be brought on by leading an unhealthy lifestyle, such as smoking and experiencing a lot of stress. Although the precise mode of transmission for H. pylori infection is still unknown, humans appear to be the only natural reservoir for the bacteria. The bacterium has been found in plaque and particularly in saliva, supporting the idea of oral transmission; nevertheless, it is unclear if the mouth is a random channel (due to vomiting or regurgitation, for example) or not.

Anti-inflammatories and other substances

Both acute and chronic gastritis can be brought on by a long-term and/or excessive use of non-steroidal anti-inflammatory drugs (NSAIDs). Abuse of these drugs can also lower the amount of a key component that protects the stomach's internal mucosa, leaving the patient more vulnerable to the development of complications. If you take them occasionally, the likelihood of stomach issues decreases.

Approximately 20% of cases of gastritis are brought on by anti-inflammatories.

In addition to anti-inflammatories, other drugs, such the following, can also cause some cases:

Alcohol

It can damage and irritate the gastric mucosa, increasing the stomach's susceptibility to digestive fluids.
Bile is a fluid that the liver produces and stores in the gallbladder. Normally, a valve keeps bile from passing from the intestine up to the stomach; however, if this valve is malfunctioning, the fluid may flow back into the stomach, resulting in inflammation and chronic gastritis.

Autoimmune gastritis

In this type of the disease, the body's defenses assault healthy stomach cells because it believes they pose a threat. Patients with various autoimmune disorders are more likely to develop autoimmune gastritis, which is more common in the elderly and usually not erosive.

Other causes

Stress

perceived as a psychosomatic response to circumstances that can promote the development of nervous gastritis, including as traumatic injuries, life-threatening diseases, severe burns, and the requirement for significant surgery. Although the precise reason for this is uncertain, it is thought to be connected to the stomach's reduced blood supply.

Coffee and spicy foods

Although there isn't any scientific proof that they can create issues at this time, it's still a good idea to stay away from them if you already have symptoms.

Incorrect lifestyle

One of the main causes of gastritis is bad behaviors, such as smoking and eating unhealthily.

Signs and symptoms

The most well-known symptoms are those of indigestion, which usually go away in a few hours. However, if they persist for several days or weeks, it's a good idea to get in touch with your health care physician. It is advisable to notify your doctor right away if you experience symptoms of gastritis after taking any particular medications. If you see blood in your vomit or feces, it's equally critical to call a healthcare provider right once (especially if the bleeding originated in the stomach, as this will result in particularly dark stools).

Common gastritis symptoms

- Bad breath
- Bitter mouth
- Stomach ache
- Weight loss
- Dysphagia
- Dyspepsia
- Hemorrhage (symptom of hemorrhagic gastritis)
- Fever (rare)
- Dark stools
- Flatulence
- Lack of appetite
- Meteorism (swollen belly)
- Nausea
- Feeling of abdominal fullness after eating
- He retched

Chronic gastritis symptoms

- Formation of ulcers
- Halitosis
- Heartburn,

- Anorexia,
- Blood in stool and vomit

Complications

Treatment for all forms of gastritis is necessary, and it can be either pharmaceutical or merely behavioral, focusing on poor lifestyle choices or eating habits. Without treatment, the symptoms of gastritis can get worse and have a serious negative impact on the patient's health. We recall the following as some of the most common consequences linked to gastritis:

- stomach sores
- stomach hemorrhage
- stomach perforations
- Possible atrophic gastritis complication: pernicious anemia
- Hyperhomocysteinemia resulting from insufficient vitamin B12, a potential side effect of atrophic gastritis

- Untreated H. pylori dependent gastritis, autoimmune atrophic gastritis complications, or an increased risk of stomach cancer
- Death and hypovolemic shock are exceedingly uncommon side effects of untreated hemorrhagic gastritis.

Additionally, a link was shown between autoimmune atrophic gastritis and several other severe conditions, including type I diabetes, thyrotoxicosis, myxedema, Addison's disease, and Hashimoto's thyroiditis.

CHAPTER 2

DIET

The first step in properly managing the condition is unquestionably paying close attention to nutrition; if gastritis or stomach acid episodes are frequent, eating lighter and more frequent meals can be quite beneficial as it lessens the consequences of gastric hyperacidity. Then, stay away from all foods that have the potential to irritate, particularly those that are fried, acidic, spicy, or greasy. Overly filling meals should also be avoided.

What to eat

- White meat (veal, turkey, rabbit, and chicken)
- Shrimp, cod, anchovies, sea bass, sea bream, and tuna fillet

- bread made with whole grains, white bread bread made with cornmeal, White rice, brown rice, Pasta
- Light spreadable cheese, lean ricotta, reduced-fat milk, mild yogurt, Cheese mozzarella
- Fruits low in citric acid, such as bananas, peaches, berries, melons, pears, and apples
- Egg
- vegetable-based fats
- veggies: potatoes, carrots, cabbage, peas, broccoli, and green beans

The recommended cooking techniques are:

- Steam-powered
- In a pressure cooker
- Boil in water
- Baked
- Grilled
- In a skillet over low heat.

What to avoid

- crimson meats
- Clams, mussels, octopus, cuttlefish, salmon, etc.
- animal fats found in hot dogs, bacon, hamburgers, and hog fat slices, among other foods.
- Garlic with onions
- Chili pepper and spices
- whole milk, sour cream dairy products high in fat, particularly fermented ones
- Potato chips, candies, or ice cream with tomatoes
- foods that have been smoked, salted, or oiled
- carbonated drinks, tea, coffee, and alcoholic beverages (particularly spirits)
- Tomato juice, white wine, peppers, sour fruit (lemons, tangerines, oranges, pineapple, currants, and pomegranates), and dried fruit (too

high in fat and protein), Coconut Vinegar

The techniques not recommended are:

- Brazing
- Frying in a pan
- Stewing

Natural cures

The dual goals of natural gastritis therapies are to lessen gastric output and shield the stomach's mucosal barrier from the harshness of acidic juices. Among the cures found in nature are the following:

CHAMOMILE

Because of its antispasmodic properties, chamomile is used to relieve abdominal pain and cramps by relaxing the muscles in the stomach. The practice of consuming a strong chamomile-based herbal tea can help prevent gastritis from reoccurring.

CABBAGE

The mucous membranes lining the digestive tract can be healed by cabbage. A glass of cabbage juice enhanced with carrot and blueberry juice, which improves the flavor and adds potent antioxidants, may help treat gastritis.

CARROT

In addition to being high in pectin, which can form a sort of gel on the stomach walls to heal them after an acid insult, carrots also contain beta carotene, which shields the mucosa against microbial attack. As a result, the precursor of vitamin A is regarded as a great natural treatment for gastritis and may help speed up the healing of ulcers.

YOGURT

Because of its emollient qualities, the potato reduces stomach inflammation and produces a nice feeling of comfort.

LICORICE

Chewing licorice pieces would be a great habit to develop in order to ease the discomfort brought on by gastritis. It is not advised to take liquorice if the patient has hypertension because large doses of the herb encourage blood pressure increases.

MAUVE

If your gastritis is accompanied by recurrent abdominal pains, an infusion based on mallow may be helpful. Mallow is a great natural cure for soothing an upset stomach.

VERDE TEA

Flavonoids, which promote healing, are the key components of tea in gastritis linked to ulcers.

CALCIUM BICARBONATE

Additional Guidance

By raising the pH of the stomach and decreasing the acidity of the gastric environment, bicarbonate helps to protect the gastric mucosa against over acidity and lessen burning. It is recommended to completely dissolve a teaspoon of baking soda in a small amount of water and drink it. Sodium bicarbonate should never be used with excessively large meals and is contraindicated in cases of hypertension.

- Increase your water intake since saliva and bodily fluids shield the esophagus muscles from stomach acids.

- Increase your intake of liquids to prevent dehydration if your gastritis symptoms are severe enough to cause vomiting and/or diarrhea. You can buy certain beverages at the pharmacy or increase your water intake; stay away from coffee and sugary drinks.
- Following a meal, taking a stroll can aid in improving digestion.

CHAPTER 3

Breakfast

1) Asparagus muffins

Ingredients:

- Asparagus 380 g
- 00 flour 250 g
- White yogurt 200 g
- Skimmed milk 200 g
- Eggs 120 g
- Parmesan 90 g
- Extra virgin olive oil 40 g
- Instant yeast for savory preparations 16 g
- Salt up to taste
- Basil to taste

Instructions

Start by removing the asparagus's hardest white portion. Trim the ends of the stems and slice the remaining halves. Halve the tips lengthwise and set them aside. Slices of asparagus should be cooked for five minutes over medium heat in a skillet with a little oil heated. Once cooked, pour the washers into a tall glass and use a hand blender to purée them into a uniform consistency. After cooking the washers for a few minutes, place the pan's tips there as well. They shouldn't fall apart, though. The tips should be moved to a small basin.

Handle the dough by adding salt to a bowl with the eggs, milk, and olive oil. After mixing with a hand whisk, add the yogurt and the yeast that has been sieved through a colander. Add the sifted flour and whisk once more to combine.

Grated cheese can be used to season the resulting mixture. Add some chopped basil leaves and the pureed asparagus to finish. Place the dough in a muffin pan. Instead of packing the molds all the way to the edge, give them some room to expand while they cook. Arrange the asparagus tips on the top and bake in a static oven that has been prepared to 200° for 20 minutes, or until the tops of the asparagus are brown. When the asparagus muffins are done, remove from the oven and allow to cool before serving.

2) Potato plumcake

Ingredients:
- Potatoes 250 g
- Flour 200 g
- Skimmed milk at room temperature 100 g
- Eggs at room temperature 175 g
- Parmesan to grate 80 g
- Water at room temperature 50 g
- Instant yeast for savory preparations 16 g
- Thyme to taste

- Salt up to 4 g
- Extra virgin olive oil as needed
- Poppy seeds to taste

Instructions

Initially, boil the potatoes for 30 to 40 minutes, or until they are cooked; the amount of time they cook will depend on their size. After cooking, reduce the potatoes to a puree by running them through a potato masher while still hot. Combine the flour, baking powder, and salt in a bowl. Add the room-temperature milk as well.

Pour the eggs and water in again. Use the electric whisk to stir the eggs until they are fully incorporated. Add the mashed potatoes that have cooled, then season with the shredded cheese and thyme leaves. After mixing and pouring the dough into a greased and oiled plum cake mold, use the back of a spoon to level the top.

Cutting the middle portion of the dough for the long side with a tiny knife that has been greased with olive oil can stop the surface from separating when cooking. Sprinkle with poppy seeds and bake on the center shelf in a static oven that has been preheated to 180° for 60 minutes. Once cooked, remove the potato plumcake from the oven, allow it to cool, and then serve.

3) Savory donut with peas and ham

Ingredients:
- Ricotta 140 g
- 00 flour 140 g
- Skimmed milk 50 ml
- Medium eggs 3
- Seed oil 25 ml
- Peas 150 g
- Sliced raw ham 100 g
- Parmesan to grate 30 g
- Instant yeast for savory preparations 1 sachet
- Salt up to taste
- Extra virgin olive oil as needed

Instructions

Add the peas to a pan with a splash of heated olive oil. Reduce the heat, stir in the water, and add the salt. Cook for a further ten minutes, stirring now and then. When ready, let it cool. Slice the ham into thin pieces.

Set aside. Pour the milk and eggs into a bowl, add the seed oil, and use a hand whisk to combine everything. Stir in the ricotta and a dash of salt. Stir in the flour, pie yeast, and grated Parmesan cheese. Blend all ingredients with a hand whisk. Add the ham and peas and stir again. Stir everything together. Pour the mixture into a 24 cm diameter donut mold that has been floured and greased, then level. Bake the donut for about 30 minutes at 180 ° in a static oven that has been prepared. Once it cools, remove the mold and serve.

4) Savory herb pancakes

Ingredients:

- Medium eggs 2
- 00 flour 100 g
- Skimmed milk 70 ml
- Swiss cheese 50 g
- 1 tbsp chopped chives
- Chopped parsley 2 tbsp
- Chopped basil 1 tbsp
- Instant yeast for savory preparations ½ tsp
- Salt up to taste
- Extra virgin olive oil (for the pan) 2 tbsp

FOR THE CREAM

- White yogurt 80 g
- 1 tbsp chopped chives
- Salt up to taste

Instructions

Once the Swiss cheese is coarsely grated, leave it aside. Chop the parsley, basil, and chives separately. Sift the flour and baking powder into a basin, then gradually add the grated cheese and chopped parsley, chives, and basil. Beat the eggs and milk in another bowl, then pour in the liquid that contains the remaining dry ingredients.

Once the mixture is smooth and soft, toss in the salt and give it one last swirl. Heat 2 tablespoons of extra virgin olive oil in a small nonstick pan over the stove. Add 3 tablespoons of dough at a time, and cook until golden on both sides of the pan. After taking the pancakes out of the pan, drain them on paper towels to keep them warm, and return the pan to the heat with another tablespoon of olive oil. Fry the remaining pancakes in the same manner. In a separate bowl, thoroughly combine the yogurt, half a teaspoon of minced chives, and salt to make the cream that will be served with the savory pancakes. Top each of the delectable herb pancakes with a tablespoon of cream and a scattering of the reserved chives before serving.

5) Yoghurt plum cake

Ingredients:
- Flour 300 g
- Eggs (about 5) 300 g
- Vegetable butter 200 g
- Low-fat yogurt 150 g
- Potato starch 50 g
- Powdered yeast 15 g
- Vanilla bean seeds 1
- Salt up to 4g

Instructions

First, fill a mixer with the following ingredients: flour, eggs, yogurt, diced butter, vanilla pod seeds, salt, yeast, and starch. For roughly three and a half minutes, work everything at maximum speed. Grease and flour a loaf pan in the interim. Transfer the mixture within as soon as it becomes homogenous. The knife blade should be dipped in melted butter before being placed in the middle of the plum cake. This will enable cooking to grow uniformly.

It is now time to cook the plumcake, which needs to be done in two stages in a static oven that has been preheated: first, for 15 minutes at 185 °C, and then for 30 minutes at 165 °C. After they are cooked, remove from the oven and allow to cool fully. Now that you've turned them out, the yogurt pancakes are prepared for tasting.

6) Milk cake

Ingredients:
- Skimmed milk 200 g
- Eggs 4
- 00 flour 200 g
- Brown sugar 180 g
- Vegetable butter 60 g
- Powdered yeast for cakes 6 g

- Organic lemon zest 1
- Salt up to 1 pinch

Instructions

Crack the eggs into a bowl, stir in a small amount of salt, and run the mixer. Stir in the sugar gradually while the mixer is running. After about ten minutes, when the mixture is frothy and clear, switch off the electric whisk. Sift the powders, flour, and yeast in a colander set over the basin. Add the ingredients gradually and stir with a spatula from bottom to top. Now take a few spoonfuls of the dough and place them in a different container. Heat the milk in a saucepan over medium heat. Add the butter and allow it to melt completely. Bring the mixture to a simmer.

Once the mixture reaches the desired temperature, remove from the heat source and transfer the mixture into the container containing the dough spoonfuls that you previously removed.

Combine thoroughly with a whisk to create a sort of batter. Proceed to transfer the batter into the bigger container containing the remaining dough, blend gently using a spatula, and then finely grate in the lemon zest. Pour the mixture into a 20 cm diameter cake pan that has been greased and floured. Bake for about 35 minutes on the lowest level of a static oven that has been warmed to 180 degrees. Place the pan on the center shelf and cook for the next ten minutes after the first twenty-five. When the cake is done, remove it from the pan, let it cool in the oven, then put it on a wire rack to finish cooling. You can now savor your hot milk cake!

7) French brioches

Ingredients:
- Warm skimmed milk 70 ml
- Fresh brewer's yeast 13 g

- Flour 0 550 g
- Vegetable softened butter 350 g
- Eggs 6
- Salt up to 15 g
- Brown sugar 80 g
- Yolks 1

Instructions

While the brewer's yeast is starting to dissolve in the warm milk, chop the butter into small pieces and allow it to soften at room temperature. Combine the sugar, salt, and sifted flour in the bowl of a planetary mixer. Stir in the dissolved yeast in the milk. After that, add the eggs and mix on low speed for 6 to 8 minutes. Boost the speed and gradually add the softened butter, adding each piece only after the prior one has been fully absorbed. The mixture will eventually start to foam and turn a pale tint. After adding more butter until the dough is extremely soft and uniform, transfer it to a bowl, cover it with plastic wrap, and leave it to rise for about three hours in a light-lit oven. Next, knead the mixture once more, turning it over with your hands two or three times, and place it in the refrigerator, covered with plastic wrap at all times, for at least 12 hours, or until the dough has set.

The dough should now be surprisingly thin. Roll it out into a sheet that is one centimeter high by transferring it to a lightly floured pastry board. Cut dough triangles and roll each one up to the tip.

Place the ends on a parchment paper-covered drip pan and gently bend them inward. Brush the brioches with the egg yolk and milk mixture that you beat in a small bowl. Allow them to rise for an additional one to thirty hours, or until their volume has doubled. The brioches should be baked for 13 to 15 minutes at 200 ° in a preheated oven, or until the tops are golden. Your brioches are here and ready to be savored.

8) Muffin with Yogurt

Ingredients:

- Flour 0 300 g
- Eggs 4
- Brown sugar 170 g
- Low-fat yogurt 220 g
- Salt up to 1 pinch
- Powdered yeast for cakes 16 g
- Soft vegetable butter 130 g
- Lemon zest 1

Instructions

Before using the butter, make sure it is soft by letting it sit out of the refrigerator for about half an hour. Next, transfer the butter into a planetary mixer fitted with a whisk (you may also use an electric mixer for this purpose). Include the sugar and run the machine on medium speed for at least 10 minutes, or until the components take on a frothy consistency. Now add the entire eggs, one at a time, being careful to wait until each is thoroughly mixed in before adding another.

Add the grated zest of one lemon and a dash of salt. Lastly, add a small amount of yogurt and keep whisking the dough until thoroughly combined. Mix the yeast and flour in a bowl, then add the sieved powders to the dough and stir with a spatula, working your way up from the bottom. Now, cut out 12 15 by 15 cm squares of parchment paper, and line a muffin pan with them. Fill the mold with the mixture all the way to the edge. After filling each mold, place them on the low shelf of a warmed static oven and bake for 30 minutes, or until the tops of the molds turn brown. When the yogurt muffins are done, allow them to cool before adding a dollop of yogurt and serving!

9) Pancakes without butter

Ingredients:

- Low-fat white yogurt 125 g
- 00 flour 150 g
- Skimmed milk 200 g
- Eggs 1
- Powdered yeast for cakes 8 g
- Extra virgin olive oil q.s.

Instructions

To begin, transfer the egg into a bowl and whisk to beat it. Once it becomes airy and light, gradually incorporate the milk and beat in the yogurt.

Then add the flour and baking powder, straining it first.

In order to avoid disassembling the mixture, continue to stir slowly and gently from the bottom to the top until you have a smooth and homogenous batter. After covering with cling film, put it in the refrigerator to rest for half an hour. Recover the batter at this point and preheat a nonstick pan over medium heat with a drizzle of oil. Place a tablespoon of batter in the middle of the pan and allow it to spread on its own. When tiny bubbles appear on the surface after a few minutes, it's time to flip the pancake with a spatula. After cooking it for a minute more, transfer it to a platter. This should be done until all of the batter is used. Serve your pancakes without butter with honey on top!

10) Apple biscuits

Ingredients:
- Apples 200 g
- Flour 250 g
- Yolks 2
- Salt up pinch 1
- Lemon zest 1
- Vegetable butter (cold from the fridge) 125 g
- Brown sugar 20 g

Instructions

Place the flour into a mixer and then add the chilled, chopped butter. Turn on the mixer and let it run until you get a sandy mixture. Spoon the mixture onto a pastry board. Add the two egg yolks and a dash of salt to the traditional fountain. Incorporate the grated lemon zest and work the dough quickly, avoiding overheating the ingredients until a dense dough is achieved. Place a fresh, dry cloth over the dough and leave it to rest. In the meantime, cut the apples into half-centimeter-sized slices and then cubes. Using a rolling pin, roll out the pastry and evenly distribute the apple chunks over the whole surface. Incorporate the apple cubes thoroughly into the crust by thoroughly mixing everything.

As you work the dough, it will warm up and get wetter; thus, as you knead it, add additional 50 grams of flour to help compact the dough again. Form your dough into the shape of a sausage, cover it with clingfilm, and refrigerate for one hour. Once this period has passed, take the sausage out of the refrigerator, unwrap it from the film, and set it aside on a chopping board. Cut into 1 centimeter-thick discs using a knife. You should get roughly twenty dosages with them.

To make the sugar grains stick to the surface, carefully press one side of each cookie into the bowl of brown sugar. Place the biscuits evenly spaced on a baking tray lined with parchment paper. Bake for 20 to 25 minutes at 180 degrees Celsius, or until the sugar has lightly crusted and the biscuits have taken on color.

Your apple cookies are now ready to be enjoyed; simply remove them from the oven and allow them to cool before serving.

11) Biscuits with olive oil

Ingredients:
- Flour 280 g
- Extra virgin olive oil ml
- Brown sugar 100 g

- Eggs 2
- Baking powder for cakes 10 g
- Salt up to 1 pinch
- Lemon zest 1
- Vanilla bean 1
- Yolks 1

Instructions

Place the whole eggs and yolk into a bowl and beat with the sugar for one minute. Add the extra virgin olive oil and the flavors (vanilla pod seeds and lemon zest) while still beating. After sifting the flour and yeast together in a bowl, add the salt, the egg, and the sugar mixture, and begin kneading. Once all the ingredients have been combined and the dough is smooth and uniform, cover it with cling film and refrigerate for at least 30 minutes. After the allotted time, lay out the dough on a floured pastry board until it is half a centimeter thick. Next, form the dough into 5 cm-diameter rounds and set them on a parchment paper-lined baking sheet.

Bake for approximately 15 minutes at 180°
in a prepared static oven. After baking,
remove the cookies from the oven, allow
them to cool fully, and then store them in
an airtight container or tin box with a lid.

12) Gluten free sponge cake

Ingredients:
- Eggs 5
- Brown sugar 150 g
- Vanilla bean 1
- Corn starch gluten free 150 g

Instructions

To make the mixture foamy, puffy, and
light yellow, start by putting the eggs in a
planetary mixer, then add the sugar and
beat the ingredients for at least 10 to 15
minutes. Once the mixture is thoroughly
whipped, feel free to add the split vanilla
pod seeds and whisk for an additional few

seconds to thoroughly blend and enhance the flavor of the combination. The starch (or potato starch) that you previously carefully sieved can now be added. Using a wooden spoon, stir everything together until the mixture is homogeneous, being cautious not to break it up. After using starch to grease and flour a 24 cm circular pan, transfer the dough to the center of the mold and smooth it out thoroughly. In a preheated static oven, bake the gluten-free sponge cake for 35 to 40 minutes at 180 ° C. Do not open the oven during the first 30 minutes of baking. Before opening, take the mold out of the oven and let the sponge cake cool inside.

CHAPTER 4

Appetizers, side dishes and snack

1) Watermelon and goat cheese finger food

Ingredients:
- Watermelon baby variety 200 g
- Goat cheese 160 g
- Chives to taste
- Salt up to taste
- Extra virgin olive oil q.s.

Instructions

Starting with the watermelon, slice it into about 3-cm-thick pieces after removing the cap. Make cuts for each slice about 3 cm apart from one another; repeat in the opposite manner to form cubes. After removing the peel, collect your cubes and use a little digger to hollow out each one. Combine the goat cheese, extra virgin olive oil, and salt in a bowl. Next, add the chopped chives (choosing the greenest, most aromatic section) and stir everything together. When the cream is uniform, stuff a tuft of goat cream into each cube, top with additional chopped chives to taste, and serve your finger feast!

2) Asparagus rolls

Ingredients:
- Asparagus 16
- Phyllo dough 2 sheets
- Salt up to taste

Instructions

Take the asparagus, rinse them, dry them with a clean cloth, cut the white base, and remove the thinnest part of the stem with the vegetable peeler. In a pot full of boiling salted water, immerse them and let them cook for 5 minutes. When they are ready, drain them in a bowl of water and ice and leave them like this for a minute: in this way, cooking will stop, and the color will not fade. Now unroll the phyllo dough and use only two sheets, overlap them and cut with a knife; you will get 16 rectangles of the same size. Drain the asparagus and dry them well with absorbent paper, then arrange the asparagus in each of the rectangles of phyllo paper and wrap. Arrange parchment paper on the lined pan and continue like this with all the others. Bake them in a static oven, already hot at 200 °, for about 15 minutes, and they will be ready to be served

3) Rolls of zucchini and shrimp

Ingredients:
- Zucchini 160 g
- Shrimp 12 (clean)
- Breadcrumbs 80 g
- 1 sprig parsley
- Extra virgin olive oil 2 tbsp
- Salt up to taste

Instructions

Slice the zucchini into 12 thin pieces after washing and trimming the ends. Lastly, chop the parsley, which you will need for the bread and the flavored oil.

Transfer the oil into a tiny bowl, stir with a teaspoon of finely chopped parsley, coat the shrimp with the infused oil, and season with salt. To prepare the breading, place the breadcrumbs in a basin, then stir in the salt and two tablespoons of finely chopped parsley. To assemble the rolls, take a slice of zucchini, put a shrimp on one end, and roll the entire thing to the other end. Finally, coat the roll in the seasoned breadcrumbs and lay it on a baking tray covered with parchment paper. baker. When all the rolls are finished, proceed with the remaining ingredients in the same manner. Season with a drizzle of oil and bake for 12 minutes at 200 ° in a static oven that has been preheated. Serve your zucchini and shrimp rolls right away after they're ready!

4) Chia seed biscuits

Ingredients:

- Eggs 8
- 00 flour 250 g
- Vegetable butter 250 g
- Potato starch 125 g
- Parmesan to grate 125 g
- Chia seeds 80 g

Instructions

Initially, bring a pot of cold water to a boil and cook the eggs for 8 minutes. After draining, allow them to cool, and then peel them. Just the yolks should be taken at this time; the egg whites won't be used for this dish. Cube the cold butter and put it in a mixer with blades; add the flour and starch and mix everything together until a crumbly consistency is achieved.

Next, include the chia seeds, firm egg yolks, and Parmesan cheese. Once more, blend everything until the ingredients are well blended. Next, place the dough on a surface dusted with flour and knead it for several minutes. Next, cover it with cling film. Refrigerate it for a minimum of forty minutes.

Next, take the dough and roll it out on a lightly floured board. You must acquire a thickness of one centimeter. Cut the cookies with a pastry cutter (5 cm in diameter) and arrange them on a parchment paper-lined drip pan.

Chia seed biscuits should be baked on the low shelf of a preheated static oven at 180 degrees for around 25 to 28 minutes. After baking, remove from the oven and allow the biscuits to cool before transferring them to a tray.

5) Croutons of bread with rosemary lentil cream

Ingredients:
- Bay leaf 2 leaves
- Vegetable broth 400 ml
- Cloves 3

- Juniper berries 3
- Extra virgin olive oil 3 tbsp
- Salt up to taste
- Dried lentils 200 g

FOR 10 CROUTONS

- Vegetable Butter 80 g
- Baguette 10 slices
- 1 sprig rosemary

Instructions

Fry the cloves, juniper berries, and bay leaves in a little oil over low heat in a nonstick pan. Stir in the dried lentils after two minutes. Cook everything on low heat for a few minutes at a time. Wet the lentils with the stock and cook, covered, for at least 45 to 60 minutes. Make frequent checks to ensure the legumes don't dry out too much; if they do, add a few ladles of broth. When the lentils are cooked, put them in a mixer, reserve a small amount for the last garnish, reduce them to a cream, and then melt half of the recipe's butter in a nonstick skillet. To make the cream more fluid, add the chopped rosemary, lentil cream, and a small amount of water to the melted butter. Stir everything well, taking care not to allow the mixture dry out too much. In another pan, toast the croutons for a few minutes, flipping them over, while slicing the bread and melting the remaining butter. Now spread the lentil cream onto each crouton. Using a teaspoon and a few rosemary needles, garnish with a small amount of the reserved lentils.

6) Steamed aromatic meatballs

Ingredients:
- Minced veal 600 g
- Water 1.5 l
- Stale bread crumb 50 g
- Vegetable broth 50 ml
- Eggs 2
- Thyme 20 sprigs
- Laurel 3 leaves
- Chives 5 g

- Parsley 5 g
- Marjoram 5 g
- Salt up to taste

Instructions

Begin chopping the aromatic herbs: use a knife to finely chop the marjoram, thyme, parsley, and chives and set them aside. Take the stale bread, scrape off the crust, chop the crumb finely in a mixer after cutting it into cubes. Pour the water and bay leaf into a big pot fitted with a steaming basket. In a bowl, beat the eggs and add the salt. Place the minced meat, the previously beaten eggs, and the mixer-chopped crumb in a separate bowl.

Mince all the ingredients together until the mixture is smooth and well-composed: chives, parsley, thyme, marjoram. In order to ensure homogenous cooking, attempt to shape some meatballs that are roughly the same size and weigh around 20 g apiece. Secure the meatballs with toothpicks, bring the water to a boil in the pot, and then remove from the heat. Put the flavorful meatballs in the steamer and simmer, covered, for about eighteen minutes. (If preferred, you can also cook the meatballs in the oven by putting them in an oiled baking dish and cooking at 180 ° for 30 minutes in a static oven or approximately 25 minutes in a convection oven at 160 °). Serve the hot, aromatic steam-cooked meatballs hot, accompanied if desired by a crisp salad.

7) Quinoa morsels

Ingredients:
- Quinoa 150 g
- Small zucchini 2
- Eggs 1
- Parmesan to be grated 50 g
- Fresh ginger to grate to taste
- Salt up to taste

Instructions

To begin, put the quinoa in a bowl and run cold water over it until the water turns clear. Next, cook the quinoa for the duration recommended on the package (about 15 to 20 minutes) in a nonstick pan with salted water, or until the grains have absorbed the majority of the cooking liquid and are soft and swollen.

To stop the quinoa from cooking, drain it and rinse it in cold water. Peel and wash the zucchini gently at this point. Next, peel and wash the fresh ginger. Grate the zucchini and add the freshly grated ginger to a big basin. Combine the egg, grated Parmesan, and the boiling quinoa with the grated zucchini in the ginger. Add salt to taste and stir the items until they are well combined. You can alternatively use a non-stick mini muffin pan. Next, place the small paper cups (about 4-5 cm in diameter and about 3 cm high) on a baking sheet and fill them with the mixture.

Using the back of a spoon, compact the mixture into the cups to better define the shape of the morsels. All you need to do is bake them for 25 minutes at 180 ° in a preheated oven (or 20 minutes at 160 ° in a convection oven) or until the tops have a nice browning. The quinoa morsels are now prepared and should be served warm!

8) Roast Potato Towers

Ingredients:

- Rosemary to taste
- Extra virgin olive oil 12 tbsp
- Potatoes 5 (about 130 gr each)
- Salt to taste

Instructions

After giving the potatoes a thorough peel, cut them into comparatively thin slices (approximately 3 mm). When slicing the potatoes, take care to keep them straight and as round and uniform as you can. Using a mixer, finely chop the rosemary and begin assembling the turrets. Season the first potato slice with salt and a pinch of chopped rosemary, then overlap the second slice and season with salt and rosemary once more. Continue this process until you have formed some "towers" that are about 4 cm high. Once all of them are prepared, put them on a baking paper-covered dripping pan and brush each turret with a tablespoon of extra virgin olive oil.

Bake everything for 25 to 30 minutes at maximum power in your oven, or until golden brown (watch out not to burn the potatoes too much). Serve the roasted potato towers straight out of the oven.

9) Baked rice croquettes

Ingredients:
- Rice 500 g
- Extra virgin olive oil 30 g
- 1L vegetable broth

FOR BREADING
- Breadcrumbs 200 g
- Eggs (medium) 4
- Salt up to taste

FOR THE STUFFING:

- Raw ham 220 g
- Peas 180 g
- Mozzarella 150 g

Instructions

In the pot, toast the rice for a short while. When the rice absorbs the liquids which should take 20 minutes or so add the broth. Once done, remove from the heat. Using a spatula, transfer the risotto to a big pan, spread it evenly, and then cover with plastic wrap to allow it to cool. Cut the ham into cubes in the interim. In addition to cutting the mozzarella into cubes, steam the peas for two minutes. Once the rice is cold, divide it into 26 equal sections, each weighing 50 g. Take one of the portions, flatten it slightly with your hands to form an oval shape, and then stuff the middle with the mozzarella, ham, and peas. Next, use the rice to enclose the croquettes, giving them an extended form. The croquettes are breaded by dipping them in the beaten egg and then the breadcrumbs. Continue in the same manner, dipping the croquette that has previously been seasoned in egg and then breadcrumbs. At this time, transfer the croquettes to a baking dish and drizzle some extra virgin olive oil over them. Preheat a static oven to 200 °C. Bake the croquettes for 30 to 35 minutes, or until golden brown. To keep the crispness of the baked rice croquettes, serve them hot.

10) Baked Pumpkin flowers

Ingredients:
- Zucchini flowers 12
- Ricotta 400 g
- Oregano to taste
- Salt up to taste
- Extra virgin olive oil as needed
- Breadcrumbs 20 g
- Grated cheese 20 g

Instructions

Transfer the ricotta cheese into a colander set over a small bowl. Use a spatula to sift the cheese to a finer consistency. Oregano-flavored and then salted.

Next, whisk together all the ingredients. It's time to clean the zucchini blossoms. Start by cutting off the stalk and removing the leaves from the base of the bloom. Blow into the blossom and use a soft brush to carefully remove any remaining earth residue. If the interior pistil is still yellow, leave it in place; if it has become too dark, remove it. Your zucchini flowers are now ready to be filled. Fill them almost to the brim, then cover them with the tops and secure them by wrapping the tips. Place the filled zucchini blossoms on a baking sheet covered with parchment paper. Place the breadcrumbs and shredded cheese in a small bowl and stir to combine the bread. Now drizzle some olive oil over the flowers, spread the bread with a spoon, and then drizzle some more olive oil over them. Bake the zucchini flowers for 7-8 minutes at 240° in a preheated oven. After cooking, remove the zucchini blossoms from the oven and allow them to cool before serving!

11) Baked potato balls

Ingredients:
- Potatoes 800 g
- Parmesan to grate 40 g
- Breadcrumbs 60 g
- Eggs 1
- Parsley 1 bunch
- Oregano 4 leaves
- Dried thyme q.s.
- Salt up to taste

FOR BREADING
- Breadcrumbs 120 g
- Eggs 2
- Extra virgin olive oil 2 tbsp

Instructions

Boil the potatoes for thirty to forty minutes first. After the parsley has been cleaned and dried, chop it. Using a potato masher, pass the potatoes with their skin on while they are still hot, and then transfer the puree to a bowl. Incorporate the parsley that has been cut, few oregano leaves, grated Parmigiano, thyme, and salt and pepper. After thoroughly mixing everything, add the egg and breadcrumbs. To create a homogenous mixture, stir. Next, form the meatballs by gently pressing them between your palms and placing them onto a platter. Get the breading ready: Beat the eggs in a basin and transfer the breadcrumbs to a different dish. Subsequently, transfer the meatballs into the egg and finally the breadcrumbs. Place every meatball onto a parchment paper-lined baking sheet, sprinkle with two teaspoons of oil, and bake at 180 °C for fifteen minutes, or until golden brown. Remove the baked potato balls from the oven when they have finished cooking and serve them hot!

12) Breaded sandwich

Ingredients:

- Mozzarella 200 g
- Eggs 2
- Salt up to taste
- Loaf bread 140 g (8 slices)
- Skimmed milk 50 g
- Breadcrumbs to taste

Instructions

Slice the mozzarella after cutting off the bread's edges. For the mozzarella to retain its liquid content during cooking, it needs to be thoroughly dried. Whisk together the salted eggs in another basin. Place a slice of bread on top of the mozzarella slices, then cover with another slice to resemble a sandwich. Pour the milk into a basin, submerge the sandwich in it, then coat it with the beaten eggs and breadcrumbs, making sure to coat the bread's sides and surface thoroughly. You can carry on with the cooking: Place the pieces to be cooked on a baking pan lined with parchment paper, and bake in a preheated oven set to 200° for 15 minutes in static mode. After the pan is done, remove it from the oven and serve it hot and stringy.

CHAPTER 5

Fish and Seafood

1) Salad rolls stuffed with tuna

Ingredients:
- Tuna fillet 100 g
- Lettuce 4 leaves
- Broad beans 400 g
- Extra virgin olive oil 40 g
- Basel 3 leaves
- Salt up to taste
- Low-fat yogurt 20 g
- Chopped pistachios to taste
- Chives 8 strands

Instructions

After shelling the beans and gathering them in the glass of the mixer, add the olive oil and blend until a cream forms. Add the yogurt and salt as well, and blend with a spoon. Smell the leaves in your palms, the cream with the minced basil.

For a few minutes, brown the tuna in a pan with a sprinkle of oil. After giving the lettuce leaves a good wash under running water, pat them dry with a cloth. Each leaf should be cut in half, being careful to remove the stiffer center. Spoon the bean and yogurt cream on half of the lettuce leaf, then load the entire leaf with chunks of cooked tuna.

The leaf should be rolled up and sealed with a chives thread. Add chopped pistachios as a garnish to taste, and repeat with the remaining ingredients.

You can now serve your tuna-filled salad wraps to the guests.

Serve them with an additional dollop of broad bean cream!

2) Cod with yogurt and purple potatoes

Ingredients:
- Cod 400 g
- Natural white yogurt 120 g

- Purple potatoes 200 g
- Extra virgin olive oil 60 g
- Salt up to taste
- Thyme to taste
- 4 slices bread
- Vegetable butter 40 g

Instructions

Place the cod fillets in a pot and boil for approximately 10 minutes, or until they become soft and white. After pouring the potatoes into cold water, boil them for approximately fifteen minutes. Drain and peel them after that. The fish and purple potatoes, peeled and roughly chopped, should be added to a blender along with extra virgin olive oil, salt, and mixing. Continue to run the mixer as you add the white yogurt and continue until the cream is creamy and whipped. Add the leaves of thyme.

Place the mixture in the refrigerator for ten to fifteen minutes or longer. Slice four pieces of bread, then apply butter over each slice. Place the slices on a baking paper-lined drip pan and toast them in a static oven prepared to 200 degrees for about ten minutes, or until golden brown. Top the toasted bread with your velvety fish mousse, purple potatoes, and yogurt. Garnish with a few thyme leaves.

3) Tuna cheesecake

Ingredients:
- Natural tuna fillets 200 g
- Light spreadable cheese 200 g
- Bread crumbs 100 g
- Vegetable butter 120 g
- Extra virgin olive oil 30 g
- Chives a few stems
- Salt up to taste

Instructions

To make crumbs, put the bread crumbs in the mixer and pulse to mix them. Bread crumbs should be added to a hot, nonstick pan and toasted for a few minutes until they turn brown. Now, use a bain-marie or microwave to melt the butter. Then, pour the butter mixture over the bread crumbs, swirl to combine, and transfer a few tablespoons of the crumbs into a pastry ring with a diameter of 9 cm. Apply pressure on the base firmly using the spoon's back. For at least fifteen minutes, place the foundation in the refrigerator to harden.

Meanwhile, make the cream: fill the mixer with the cheese, tuna, and chives; add the olive oil, salt, and blend until the mixture is smooth. After the base has solidified, pour the cream over the entire piece of bread, smoothing it out with the back of a teaspoon. Place back in the fridge for ten minutes to solidify. After the cream has solidified as well, remove the cheesecakes and top them with some tuna chunks before adding some chives for flavor. It's time to serve the tuna cheesecake.

4) Cod and ham morsels

Ingredients:

- Cod fillet 300 g
- Sliced raw ham 100 g
- Bread (crumb) 30 g
- 1 sprig rosemary
- 1 sprig parsley
- Chives to taste
- Salt up to 1 pinch
- Extra virgin olive oil as needed

Instructions

Prepare the chopped herbs and place them in a bowl with the breadcrumbs that have been crumbled. Cut the fish fillets into small, but not tiny, cubes. Drizzle some oil into a skillet, bring to a simmer, then add the fish. Allow to brown on all sides, rotating occasionally, for a total of five minutes. Add the salt last, then move the mixture to a platter. After that, run the cod cubes through the breading until completely covered. Arrange the ham slices on a chopping board, starting with the first slice of each codpiece. To get a roll, roll up. Repeat with the remaining ones and transfer to an ovenproof dish. Bake for ten minutes at 180 ° in a static oven that has been prepared. After that, take it out of the oven and let it cool. Place a little bowl and some lettuce leaves on a platter, then add the morsels. You may now serve your cod bites!

5) Honey roasted shrimp

Ingredients:
- Shrimp (Clean) 36
- Honey 100 g
- Fresh ginger 3 g
- Salt up to taste
- FOR THE FAKE MAYONNAISE
- Sunflower oil 100 ml
- Soy milk 50 ml
- Mint 8 leaves
- Salt up to taste

Instructions

Grate and peel the raw ginger. Add the honey, ginger, and eight pinches of salt to a pot. Cook for five minutes on medium heat to heat and thicken. Allow the sauce to cool. Assemble the skewers now, putting three shrimp on each wooden skewer. Put aside and make the imitation mayonnaise by combining the milk, mint leaves, and seed oil in a tall, narrow bowl. Using the immersion blender, mix in salt until a smooth cream is achieved. After that, you may continue cooking by brushing the skewers with the honey sauce and grilling them for a few minutes on each side over a hot grill. Serve the honey-roasted skewers with the imitation mint mayonnaise on the side.

6) Sole in the pan

Ingredients:
- Clarified butter 120 g
- flour q.s.

- 1 sprig parsley
- Salt up to taste
- Skimmed milk to taste
- Medium sole 4 (clean)

Instructions

After dipping the sole in the milk, both sides should be coated in flour. After that, put them in a skillet with clarified butter and fry them for 3 to 4 minutes on each side, or until they are golden brown. When turning them, take extreme caution to avoid breaking the soles! Meanwhile, use a knife to finely chop the parsley. Once the sole is cooked, season with salt and freshly chopped parsley.

Garnish the solitary dish with parsley sprigs and serve right away!

7) Tuna with sesame

Ingredients:
- Tuna (4 fillets) 150 g
- Black sesame seeds 10 g
- White sesame seeds 20 g

- Extra virgin olive oil 35 g
- Lemon juice 25 g
- Salt up to taste

Instructions

Transfer the sesame seeds to a plate and stir to combine. Regarding the tuna, we advise you to confirm that it has been slaughtered before purchasing it. It is also advised that you freeze it for a minimum of 96 hours at -18 degrees Celsius, and then thaw it out before utilizing the recipe. To ensure that the seeds are properly toasted on both sides, pass the tuna slices over them. When a non-stick pan is hot, add the breaded tuna fillets and fry over high heat for one minute. Then, flip them over with a spatula and cook for an additional minute. The tuna will be raw inside once it has been seared, but you can cook it longer if you'd like. After cooking, place the fillets on a chopping board, cut them into slices right away, and serve right away.

CHAPTER 6

Meat

1) Salad baskets with turkey

Ingredients:
- Turkey breast 250 g
- Baby lettuce 100 g
- Cashews 25 g
- Carrots 1
- Parsley to taste
- Extra virgin olive oil q.s.

Instructions

On a chopping board, arrange the turkey breast and cut it into asymmetrical pieces. Then, heat a thin layer of oil in a nonstick pan. Add the salt and the turkey breast pieces. Cook the morsels inside for approximately 10 minutes, flipping them occasionally, until they are golden brown. After the turkey morsels are cooked, put them in a mixer and run it for a few seconds to chop the flesh finely. Then, pour the combined mixture into a big bowl. Now put the cashews on a chopping board and roughly chop them. In a nonstick skillet, roast the chopped cashews for a few minutes until they become crunchy and darker. Next, combine the chopped turkey bites with the toasted cashews. Next, take a carrot, cut it in half, and peel it.

Cut it into little cubes after that.

In addition, rinse the parsley under running water and roughly chop it on a chopping board. At this point, include the chopped parsley and diced carrot into the mixture. After giving the salad a gentle wash, arrange the crispest and most curled leaves on a serving dish. After that, continue filling them with dough. It's time to serve your turkey and lettuce baskets.

2) Meatballs in sesame crust

Ingredients:

- Minced veal 300 g
- Wholemeal bread crumb 65 g
- Parmesan (for grating) 50 g
- Sesame seeds 50 g
- Black sesame seeds 25 g
- Eggs 1
- Salt up to taste

Instructions

After removing the outer crust, cut the wholemeal bread crumb into cubes and crush it into a mixer. Place the veal in a big basin and mix it with your hands. Next, add the grated cheese and the minced breadcrumbs. Add the egg and salt for seasoning. Using your hands, stir until a homogenous mixture is achieved. Each time you do this, you will need to obtain 38 meatballs using our doses, or until you have finished the available mix. Transfer the white sesame seeds to a plate and carefully combine them with the black sesame seeds. Make sure the sesame adheres firmly to the meat by passing the meatballs over it. Proceed with the remaining meatballs in this manner, and when you're done, place them side by side on a baking tray covered with parchment paper. If needed, season the meatballs with a drizzle of oil before baking them for about 25 minutes at 180 degrees in a static oven that has been prepared. Take the meatballs with a sesame crust out of the oven when the timer goes off and savor them hot.

3) Veal slices with mushrooms

Ingredients:
- Veal (walnut) 400 g
- Champignon mushrooms 500 g
- Vegetable butter 50 g
- 00 flour 40 g
- Extra virgin olive oil 10 g
- Salt up to taste
- Thyme to taste
- 1 sprig chopped rosemary

Instructions

After flouring the veal slices on both sides and squeezing out any excess flour, take the veal slices and thinly slice them with the meat mallet. Now take care of cleaning the mushrooms. Using a tiny knife, start to scrape off the earthy portion of the stem, gently removing any remaining dirt. If the mushroom is sufficiently clean, use a brush to remove any remaining dirt; avoid giving them a water bath to avoid contaminating them. After slicing, put the mushrooms aside. Now carry out the meat's cooking: Melt half of the butter (25 g) in a pan with the olive oil. After the butter is melted, place the floured veal slices on the pan, season with salt, and cook for 3 minutes on each side, or until a crust forms.

After they are golden brown, transfer them to a platter to cool and tend to the mushrooms: Melt the remaining half of the butter in the pan you used to cook the beef, season with the chopped rosemary, add the sliced mushrooms, and sauté them for two minutes over medium heat before adding salt. The veal slices should now be added, browned, set aside, and flavored with the thyme leaves. Cook for a minute over low heat, adding a ladle of water if needed, and serve the veal and mushrooms hot!

4) Milk chicken breasts

Ingredients:
- Sliced chicken breast 4
- Vegetable butter 40 g
- Extra virgin olive oil 10 g
- 00 flour q.s.
- Skimmed milk 170 g
- Salt up to taste
- Thyme 4 sprigs

Instructions

Lay the slices out on a chopping board and pound them with a meat mallet until the slices are very thin. Butter and oil should be slowly melted in a skillet while the chicken slices are being floured. Turn up the heat a little as you transfer them to the pan, and then give them another two minutes or so to develop a lovely crust. After flipping the slices and waiting for a few more minutes, add the milk to the pan first, followed by the thyme leaves.

After adding the salt and covering the pan, heat for an additional four to five minutes, or until the milk has thickened. All you need to do now is serve your hot, milk-filled chicken breasts!

5) Tasty chicken wings and potatoes

Ingredients:
- Chicken wings 8
- Potatoes 500 g
- Breadcrumbs 200 g
- 00 flour 50 g
- Parmesan to grate 50 g
- Eggs 2
- Parsley to be minced to taste
- Extra virgin olive oil as needed
- Salt up to taste

Instructions:

First, transfer the flour into a bowl, coat the chicken wings with it on both sides, shake off any extra, and put them on a tray. Place the breadcrumbs, grated Parmesan cheese, chopped parsley (reserving some for the finishing touch) and stir well in a separate bowl. Lastly, beat the eggs once more in a different basin. Using your hands to provide a firm hold, dip the floured chicken wings first in the beaten egg, followed by the breadcrumbs and Parmesan cheese. To ensure that the breading stays on the meat as it cooks, it is crucial to flour it beforehand. After all of the chicken wings have been breaded, you may handle the potatoes.

After peeling, cut the potatoes into quarters, then half. Afterward, cut the potatoes into cubes. After adding salt and oil to a bowl, add the potatoes to the bowl with the remaining bread and well mix.

This is the time to grab a big skillet, add the breaded chicken wings, and then equally spread the potatoes over the bottom. Add a little pinch of salt and a generous amount of oil for seasoning, then bake for 40 minutes at 200° in a preheated convection oven. To ensure that the bread is crispy, turn on the grill and cook for a further 10 minutes.

While the potatoes are still steaming and your tasty chicken wings are cooked, top with the leftover parsley!

6) Stuffed turkey rolls

Ingredients:
- Turkey breast (4 slices)
- Salt up to taste
- Seed oil 3 tbsp
- Rosemary 8 sprigs
- Scamorza 8 slices
- 8 slices raw ham

Instructions

After using a meat tenderizer to beat the slices, cover them with baking paper.

Take a piece of chicken and load it with two slices of raw ham and two slices of smoked cheese. Roll the slice in on itself. Using a wooden skewer, cut the roll in half so that it stops. Garnish each roll with a rosemary sprig for flavor. Continue this method with the remaining turkey slices.

The rolls are now prepared for grilling. Preheat a grill and coat it with a little seed oil. Cook the rolls for at least 6 or 7 minutes on each side, or until they are nicely grilled. Then, sprinkle them with salt and set them aside to cool before serving.

7) Roasted rabbit

Ingredients:
- Rabbit in pieces 1.2 kg
- Rosemary 4 sprigs
- Salt up to taste
- Vegetable broth 2000 g
- Potatoes 800 g
- Thyme 4 sprigs

- Bay leaf 1 leaf
- Extra virgin olive oil 80 g

Instructions

After chopping the rosemary, put half of it in a skillet with 40 grams of oil in it. Simmer it for two to three minutes on low heat with a bay leaf added. Turn up the heat and add the rabbit pieces. Cook for three to four minutes on each side. Cook for a further five to six minutes over low heat after adding a ladle of broth. Prepare the potatoes in the meanwhile by peeling and chopping them into fairly big pieces. Place all the ingredients in a basin, season with the chopped rosemary needles, and reserve the salt and thyme leaves.

Add 20 grams of oil and stir. After transferring everything to a sizable pan, evenly distribute the potatoes using roughly 10 g of oil. Next, lay the pieces of previously browned rabbit as well. Cook the rabbit and potatoes together in a static oven that has been set to 200° for 40 minutes, then add the remaining vegetable broth. Serve your rabbit when it's still steaming in the oven after taking it out!

8) Chicken meatloaf

Ingredients:
- Minced chicken 800 g
- Swiss cheese 150 g
- Ricotta 100 g
- Parmesan to grate 50 g
- Eggs 1
- Breadcrumbs 70 g
- Marjoram 3 sprigs
- Extra virgin olive oil 10 g
- Salt up to taste

Instructions

Cut the cheese into cubes first, then put them in a blender and combine everything together. Move the chicken mince to a bowl and mix in the egg, grated cheese, marjoram leaves, well-drained ricotta, and marjoram leaves. Mix the ingredients with your hands until smooth, then add the breadcrumbs and knead once more. Transfer the mixture onto a piece of parchment paper, using your hands to form it into a meatloaf shape. Next, enclose the loaf in the same parchment paper and secure it tightly. Put the container in the fridge for a minimum of one hour to solidify. After that, take off the parchment paper and preheat the oil in a big pot or pan that can be baked in the oven.

With two stirrers or kitchen tongs, brown the meatloaf on all sides to create a lovely crust and prevent it from splitting. At this point, bake the pan in static mode for 60 minutes at 200° with the foil covered.

After cooking, remove your chicken meatloaf from the oven and serve it with a sprinkle of its cooking juices (if you have a thermometer, make sure the internal temperature has reached 70 to 71 degrees).

9) Turkey chunks with saffron

Ingredients:

- Turkey breast 600 g
- Saffron (one sachet) 0.15 g
- Water about 140 g
- Extra virgin olive oil 10 g
- Potato starch 1 tsp
- flour q.s.
- Salt up to taste

FOR THE ASPARAGUS

- Asparagus 400 g
- Water 100 g
- Extra virgin olive oil 10 g
- Salt up to taste

CHAPTER 7

Unique dishes

1) Lentil pie

Ingredients:
- Potatoes 400 g
- Lentils 100 g
- Spinach 400 g
- Eggs 1
- Mozzarella 50 g
- Parmesan 50 g
- Breadcrumbs 40 g
- Vegetable butter 50 g
- Extra virgin olive oil 30 g
- Salt up to taste

Instructions

Wash the spinach first. Heat the oil in a big skillet, add the slightly wet spinach, season with salt, and cook, stirring occasionally with a wooden spoon, for around five minutes. Lastly, drain and remove from the heat. After peeling, chop the potatoes into cubes. Transfer the potatoes to a pot of boiling water. After draining and rinsing, add the lentils to the pot with the potatoes. Add the salt and cover and simmer for approximately 20 minutes. After that, rinse the veggies and transfer them to a bowl. Using a fork, mash the potatoes and lentils until a creamy puree is achieved. Mix with 30 grams of butter. Stir one more and add the egg after adding the Parmesan. Blend thoroughly.

Cut mozzarella into square pieces. Using a pastry brush, grease eight disposable aluminum molds with ten grams of melted butter, then dust them with breadcrumbs. Partially fill each mold with the lentils and mashed potatoes.

Next, add some cooked spinach and/or diced mozzarella. Finally, use the back of a spoon to press down on the lentil and potato mixture to cover. Add a generous amount of breadcrumbs. Place a small piece of butter on the surface and bake for about 30 minutes in static mode on the middle shelf of an oven that has been set to 180 °C. The golden pies should be taken out of the oven, turned over, and served hot.

2) Baskets of potatoes with zucchini and cheese

Ingredients:
- Potatoes 300 g
- Zucchini 200 g
- Mozzarella g
- Extra virgin olive oil as needed
- Salt up to taste
- Oregano to taste

Instructions

After peeling, thinly slice the potatoes (to a thickness of 1 mm). After transferring them to a bowl, season with oregano, salt, and olive oil. After thoroughly flavoring, grease 12 aluminum molds and lay the potato slices so that they completely cover the molds, starting from the bottom and working their way up to the inner edges. Now put them on a rack in the oven and cook for 20 minutes at 200° in a convection oven that has been preheated. Meanwhile, wash and trim the zucchini, then cut them into cubes. Meanwhile, cut the mozzarella into cubes. Add the oil to a skillet, add the zucchini, season with salt, and cook over medium heat for 15 minutes. Once cooked, set aside. After the baskets are done cooking, remove them from the oven. Place a few mozzarella cubes within the baskets, followed by the zucchini and a final layer of mozzarella. Return it to the oven for ten minutes at this time, just long enough to melt the mozzarella. After turning the potato baskets over and allowing them to cool a little, serve them from the table.

3) Chickpea crepes with cod mousse

Ingredients

- Chickpea flour 100 g
- Water 250 g
- Extra virgin olive oil 1 tbsp
- Salt up to 1 pinch

FOR THE COD MOUSSE

- Cod 600 g
- Skimmed milk 300 g
- Ricotta 100 g
- Sage 1 leaf
- Bay leaf 1 leaf
- Parsley 5 g
- Chives to taste
- Salt up to 1 pinch

Instructions

After peeling, thinly slice the potatoes (to a thickness of 1 mm). After transferring them to a bowl, season with oregano, salt, and olive oil. After thoroughly flavoring, grease 12 aluminum molds and lay the potato slices so that they completely cover the molds, starting from the bottom and working their way up to the inner edges. Now put them on a rack in the oven and cook for 20 minutes at 200° in a convection oven that has been preheated.

Meanwhile, wash and trim the zucchini, then chop it into cubes. Also chop the mozzarella into cubes. Add the oil to a skillet, add the zucchini, season with salt, and cook over medium heat for 15 minutes. Once cooked, set aside.

In the meantime, remove the baskets from the oven after they are done cooking. Place a few mozzarella cubes within the baskets, followed by the zucchini and a final layer of mozzarella. Return it to the oven for ten minutes at this time, just long enough to melt the mozzarella. After removing the potato baskets and allowing them to cool somewhat, place them on the table for serving.

4) Shrimp omelette

Ingredients:
- Medium eggs 8
- Shrimp 800 g (Clean)
- Parsley 4 sprigs
- Extra virgin olive oil 20 g
- Salt up to taste

Instructions

After cleaning, gently dry the parsley stalks with a paper towel or clean kitchen towel. After that, transfer them to a chopping board and coarsely chop. The eggs should now be broken into a basin, beaten with a fork or whisk, and salted to taste. Heat some oil in a nonstick skillet, add the parsley, and cook for a short while. After the prawns have been washed and shelled, add them to the sauce and cook over medium heat for around five minutes, or until they start to turn pink. Following this, pour the whisked eggs into the pan, turning it to ensure the mixture coats the entire surface. Reduce the heat to low and cook for 2 minutes. Then, cover and cook for an additional 5 to 6 minutes, or until the surface thickens enough. At this point, flip the omelet over and slide it back into the pan using the cover or a plate, then cook for a further two minutes on the other side without a lid. Turn off the heat and serve your shrimp omelet hot or cold once it has a thicker consistency and a deeper color!

5) Potato pie in a pan

Ingredients:
- Potatoes (about 1) 180 g
- Parmesan to grate 40 g
- Zucchini flowers 6
- Mozzarella 100 g
- Raw ham 100 g

Instructions

To keep the potatoes from going black, first wash and pat dry them in their skins. Then, thinly slice them and put them in a bowl of water. Cut the stem off of the zucchini flowers and separate the leaves from the flower base. Gently brush out any remaining soil from inside the blossom. Split the bloom open and extract the pistil. Cube the mozzarella and set it aside. After draining and patting dry the potato slices, heat a nonstick pan and add the first layer of potatoes on the spiral bottom. After forming a circle, lay the potatoes overlapping each other, and then insert a potato in the center to ensure that there are no spaces between the slices.

Distribute a portion of the cheese over the entire area. After placing the lid on, heat for two to three minutes. As before, arrange more potatoes in a spiral pattern. Next, cover the whole surface with a layer of cheese. Add half of the sliced ham, half of the zucchini flowers, and even half of the mozzarella cubes to the cavity now. Proceed by adding the remaining uncooked ham and zucchini flowers, covering them with extra cheese and mozzarella cubes.

After placing the lid on, simmer everything for around ten minutes. To appreciate the potato pie's racy flavor, serve it in the pan right away!

6) Saffron risotto

Ingredients:
- Saffron in pistils 1 tsp
- Rice 320 g
- Vegetable butter 125 g
- Parmesan cheese to be grated 80 g
- Water q.s.
- Vegetable broth 1 l
- Salt up to taste

Instructions

To release the color of the saffron pistils, first place them in a small glass, cover the pistils fully with water, stir, and then allow the mixture to infuse for the entire night. Next, make the vegetable broth (one liter is needed for the dish). Pour 50g of the appropriate amount of butter into a large skillet, melt it over low heat, add the rice, and toast it for 3-4 minutes to allow the grains to seal and continue cooking.

Then cook for another 18 to 20 minutes, covering the grains the entire time and adding the liquid a ladle at a time as needed as the rice absorbs it. Pour the water infused with the saffron pistils five minutes before the cooking process ends and mix. Once cooked, remove from the heat, toss in the salt, grated cheese, and the remaining 75 grams of butter, stir, cover, and set aside to rest for a few minutes. The saffron risotto is now prepared; serve it hot.

7) Cream of cauliflower

Ingredients:
- Cauliflower 740 g
- Potatoes and 740 g
- Salt up to taste
- Extra virgin olive oil 3 tbsp

- Chives stem 1
- Vegetable butter 30 g
- Leeks 110 g
- Water 1 l

Instructions

Clean, peel, and chop the potatoes. Scoop off the green portion of the leek and thinly slice the white portion. After washing and cleaning the cauliflower, trim the lower end of the head with a knife, removing any tough leaves, and then separate the florets from the stem. In a saucepan, melt the butter together with two teaspoons of oil. Cook the potatoes, cauliflower, leek, and one liter of water over medium heat for ten minutes, stirring periodically. After that, cover the pot and cook on low heat for an additional twenty minutes. After the veggies are cooked, use the mixer to combine everything together. Chop the chives, sprinkle them over the cream, add salt for seasoning, and thoroughly combine all the ingredients. It's time to serve the cauliflower cream hot, maybe with some toasted bread croutons, extra virgin olive oil, and grated Parmesan cheese.

8) Risotto with apples and speck

Ingredients:
- Rice 320 g
- Apples 2
- Raw ham 120 g (sliced)
- Vegetable broth to taste
- Vegetable butter 50 g
- Parmesan 50 g
- Rosemary to taste

Instructions

Make the vegetable broth first, and then keep it heated. Next, take the ham pieces and roughly cut them. Now proceed to the apples; cut them into four pieces, then peel and chop them into cubes. To keep them from turning black, slowly submerge them in water that has been acidified. Half of the butter should be put in a pan; the remaining portion will be used to stir the risotto at a later time. After the butter has melted, add the rice. For a few minutes, toast it while stirring often. Wet the rice with the hot broth starting now and stopping only as necessary. Pour a small amount of oil into a different heated pan, add the ham and the apples, and cook over high heat. Add the ham and apples to the risotto after it has been cooking for about three minutes. Turn off the heat as soon as the rice is done cooking and sprinkle the remaining butter and Parmesan over the top. To complete stirring, cover the pan with a lid, wait one minute, stir gently, and shake the pan. When the risotto is cooked, serve it with a few rosemary needles as a garnish.

9) Cream of peas

Ingredients:
- Peas 1 kg
- Fresh liquid cream 20 g

- Grated cheese 50 g
- Extra virgin olive oil 30 g
- Salt up to taste
- Vegetable broth 400 g

Instructions

Heat the oil in a pan over low heat, add the peas and salt, and stir everything together. After cooking for roughly five minutes, pour 350 g of vegetable broth over the top. Simmer for a further 15 to 20 minutes, then remove from the heat and puree everything with an immersion blender, adding the reserved vegetable broth, until it's smooth. After adding the fresh cream, return the heat to medium and cook, stirring frequently, for an additional five minutes. To make your pea cream even creamier, transfer it to a strainer and use a spatula to sift it.

Serve your pea soup hot or lukewarm, according to your preference, and sprinkle with Parmesan, to taste!

CHAPTER 8

Dessert

1) Baked Pears

Ingredients:
- Pears 2
- Ricotta 200 g
- Spreadable cheese 80g
- Honey 40 g
- Chopped chives to taste
- Extra virgin olive oil as needed
- Salt up to taste
- Baked Pears

Instructions

Wash and dry the fruits first. Remove the core and a tiny portion of the pulp from the pears by cutting them in half lengthwise. To make the peels more comfortable to place on the pan, cut a small portion off of the side. After that, arrange them on a baking sheet covered with parchment paper and sprinkle with

salt and oil. Bake for 10 minutes, or until they are just tender, in a static oven that has been preheated to 180 degrees. After cooking, take it out of the oven and allow it to cool. Get the filling ready by combining the cream cheese, ricotta, and salt in a bowl and using an immersion mixer to blend until a smooth cream is achieved. To emulsify, add the chopped chives and honey and stir with a spoon.
Place the cream inside the cooked pears. Serve your roasted pears right away with honey and gorgonzola.

2) Apple Pie

Ingredients:
- Apples 700 g
- Brown sugar 200 g
- 00 flour 250 g
- Vegetable butter 100 g
- Skimmed milk (at room temperature) 150 g
- Eggs (at room temperature) 2

- Salt up to 1 pinch
- Baking powder
- Lemon 1

Instructions

In a double boiler or the microwave, melt the butter and set it aside. In order to keep the apples from blackening, peel, cut, and transfer them into a bowl. Sprinkle with the lemon juice and stir thoroughly. After that, sift the baking powder and 00 flour. Next, combine the eggs and a portion of the sugar in a big bowl. Pour the sugar in a bit at a time and begin beating with the electric whisk. Add a little sprinkle of salt as soon as the mixture starts to lighten, then continue whipping until it becomes fluffy and light. Add the melted butter that has been brought back to room temperature at this point. Next, add the baking powder and sifted flour one tablespoon at a time while whisking continuously.

Once the ingredients are all mixed in, reduce the speed of the electric whisk and gradually add the room temperature milk. The dough is ready when the milk is fully mixed, so stop whipping. Pour the apples into the mixture after draining them in a sieve to extract the lemon juice. Stir gently to fully incorporate, working your way up to the bottom.

Pour the ingredients into a cake pan with a 22 cm diameter after greasing and sugar-sprinkling it. The cake is prepared for baking; bake it for approximately 55 minutes at 180 ° in a static oven that has been preheated. When cooked, remove from the oven and allow to cool fully before removing from the pan. You can now enjoy your apple pie!

3) Light cheesecake

Ingredients:
- Wholemeal dry biscuits 180 g
- Light butter 80 g

FOR THE CREAM
- Light spreadable fresh cheese 500 g

- Low-fat yogurt 250 g
- Fructose 160 g
- Gelatin in sheets 10 g
- Water 30 g
- Vanilla bean 1

Instructions

Place the wholemeal biscuits in the mixer and pulse to finely chop them. Put the crumbled biscuits into a bowl. Now, heat the butter in a skillet. Slowly pour the melted butter into the bowl containing the chopped biscuits, and stir everything together thoroughly to form a sandy mixture.

Grease a 24 cm diameter cake pan; cut out two strips the same height as the sides and a disc of parchment paper the same diameter as the pan's bottom, then line. Spoon the crumbled biscuits onto the parchment paper-lined baking tray, then use a spoon to firmly press down on the biscuit foundation. Allow the mixture to cool for thirty minutes in the fridge or ten minutes in the freezer. Now focus on the filling: soak the gelatin sheets in cold water for approximately ten minutes to soften them, then squeeze them thoroughly. In the meantime, combine the fructose and spreadable cheese in a blender and use a whisk to blend the ingredients. Next, include the vanilla bean seeds. Stir in the low-fat yogurt and beat in the whips until well combined. The gelatine sheets will have sufficiently softened in the meanwhile. Once it has melted fully, dissolve it in 30 grams of boiling water in a saucepan and add it to the cheese and yogurt mixture. Using a hand whisk, thoroughly combine all the ingredients to create a creamy and homogenous mixture. The cream is now ready; spread it over the chilled, compacted biscuit base. To level out the cream, smooth it out. After that, chill your light cheesecake for at least 4 hours to solidify it, and then serve it!

4) Coconut biscuits

Ingredients:

- Rapè coconut 150 g
- Brown sugar 120 g
- Egg whites 3

Instructions:

Transfer the rapé coconut to a bowl, stir in the sugar, and then fold in the egg whites. Make sure to fully combine all the ingredients; you may need to work until the mixture is homogeneous. Next, using a spoon, take little portions of the dough and place them in a drip pan that has parchment paper on it. Bake roughly eighteen cookies. Bake for approximately 10 minutes, or until the tops are brown, at 200 ° in a convection oven that has been warmed. After removing them from the oven, allow them to cool. Once chilled, present your coconut candies!

5) Carrot treats

Ingredients:
- Carrots 250 g
- Brown sugar 200 g
- 00 flour 250 g
- Potato starch 50 g
- Eggs 1
- Yolks 1
- Seed oil 130 ml
- Orange peel 1
- Vanilla bean 1
- Powdered yeast 8 g

Instructions:

Peel and thoroughly wash the carrots before chopping them into small pieces in a blender. Beat the eggs and the sugar together in a big bowl. Add the diced carrots after the mixture is frothy and light in color. Add the flour, potato starch, and yeast to the egg and sugar mixture after sieving them. Lastly, stir in the vanilla bean seeds and orange zest. Next, thoroughly mix in the seed oil; the dough should be very soft. Pour the carrot mixture into each of the 12 muffin molds (diameter: approximately 6/7 cm) that have been lined with paper cups (or butter and flour them). Leave about a centimeter at the top of each mold. Preheat a static oven to 180 °C. Bake the patties for about 20 to 25 minutes, or until a stick inserted in the center of one comes out clean; they won't be completely dry.

Once cooled, take them out of the molds and serve.

6) Water cake

Ingredients:
- Natural water, at room temperature 330 g
- 00 flour 300 g
- Brown sugar 200 g
- Powdered yeast 16 g
- Seed oil 90 g

- Vanilla bean 1

Instructions:

First, place the flour and yeast in a basin and set it alone for a little while. Pour the sugar into a different basin, then add the room-temperature water and whisk vigorously to dissolve the sugar. Slice a vanilla pod lengthwise with a knife to extract the seeds, which you will then combine with the sugar and water. Now pour in the seed oil and stir. Now, add the sifted powders to the emulsion of water, sugar, and oil one spoon at a time, making sure to constantly mix thoroughly to prevent lumps from forming. You will have a soft, smooth, and lump-free dough after adding all of the flour. Line a 24 centimeter diameter mold with baking paper.

Alternatively, if you'd rather, you could just use a tablespoon of flour and a small amount of seed oil to oil and flour it. Pour the cake mixture into the mold when it's ready.

Preheat a static oven to 180 ° and bake for 50 minutes. After cooking the cake for 30 minutes, cover it with a sheet of aluminum foil and continue cooking if you feel that the color of the cake is too intense. Test the cake with a toothpick before removing it from the oven; if it comes out clean and dry, the cake has cooked through. Take the cake out and let it cool. You can now enjoy your water cake!

7) Soft ricotta and pear cake

Ingredients:
- Pears 400 g
- Cow's milk ricotta 350 g
- 00 flour 250 g
- Powdered yeast for cakes 16 g
- Eggs 3
- Brown sugar 170 g
- Lemon zest 1
- Vanilla bean 1

Instructions

To keep the pears from blackening, cut them into tiny cubes and place them in a basin with very little lemon juice. Add the seeds from the vanilla pod after whisking the sugar and ricotta with a whisk or in a planetary mixer. Next, add the grated lemon zest and beat in the remaining three eggs one at a time. Using a wooden spoon, stir the flour and baking powder into the mixture until a smooth dough is achieved. Add the chopped pears and stir them into the dough.

The cake dough should be added to a pan that is 24 cm in diameter, well greased and floured, and then leveled with a spatula. Now, bake the cake for 50-70 minutes at 180 °C, or until a wooden toothpick inserted in the center comes out clean. Cover the cake with aluminum foil if the top of the cake becomes overly black while cooking. Remove the soft cake with ricotta and pear from the oven, let it cool, then remove it from the mold, sprinkle it, and serve!

8) Honey cake

Ingredients:
- Honey 250 g
- 00 flour 200 g
- White yogurt 110 g
- Vegetable butter 65 g
- Potato starch 50 g
- Eggs 3
- Powdered yeast for cakes 16 g
- Orange peel 1

Instructions:

In a saucepan, gently warm the honey, then remove from the heat and stir in the yogurt and butter. Separate the yolks from the whites of the eggs and add them to the honey mixture. Using a whisk, stir the mixture until it becomes homogenous, then transfer it to a bowl. Now, sieve the flour, baking powder, cinnamon, and starch in separate batches. Mix the powders into the honey mixture, add the grated orange peel for seasoning, and put aside.

Set the oven's temperature to 200° in static mode. Next, take the reserved egg whites and use an electric whisk to beat them until they become foamy. Finally, add the mixture to the whipped egg whites and gently stir using a spatula from the bottom up. high until the mixture becomes uniform. Line a 22 cm-diameter mold with grease and flour, then pour the dough into it. The honey cake can now be baked for 40 minutes at 200° in a static oven that has been preheated.

Once cooked, remove the cake from the oven, allow it to cool, then invert and serve.

9) Sweet zucchini pie

Ingredients:
- Zucchini 300 g
- 00 flour 350 g

- Eggs 3
- Corn oil 200 ml
- Brown sugar 250 g
- Baking powder for cakes 1 sachet
- Vanilla bean 1

Instructions

Wash the zucchini, cut off the ends, and then grate them. Add the flour and the well-sifted yeast after beating the entire eggs and sugar together until the mixture is light and fluffy. They then beat the vanilla pod seeds as well. Moreover, add the seed oil and thoroughly mix it up before adding the grated zucchini last. Combine all ingredients and transfer the blend into a 24 x 26 cm pan that has been buttered and floured (or lined with parchment paper). Bake the zucchini cake at 180 °C for approximately 60 minutes. After the first 40 minutes of cooking, if the surface gets too black, cover it with aluminum foil. Before transferring the zucchini sweet cake, let it cool.

10) Peach cake

Ingredients:

- Peaches (cleaned 285 g) 330 g
- 00 flour 280 g
- Brown sugar 170 g
- Seed oil 90 g
- Skimmed milk at room temperature 90 g
- 3 eggs at room temperature 155 g
- Powdered yeast for cakes 16 g
- Lemon zest 1

Instructions

Preheat the oven to 180 degrees. Next, rinse the peaches under running water, pat dry, and chop them into fairly large pieces. 285 grams of peach pulp will be required. Weigh each ingredient carefully and add it to the mixer in the following order: peaches in wedges, sugar, flour, whole eggs, yeast, and lemon zest; liquids come last, consisting of milk and seed oil. Run the blades through everything and process until a creamy consistency is achieved.

Pour the ingredients into a cake pan with a 22 cm diameter that has been greased and floured. The dough can now be cooked. Bake for 60 minutes at 180 degrees in a preheated oven. After cooking, remove the peach pan from the oven and allow it to cool completely before slicing it.

11) Yogurt smoothie

Ingredients:
- Low-fat yogurt 250 g
- Lime juice (about 1) 13 g
- Pulp melon 420
- Peaches pulp 350 g

Instructions

To make the yogurt smoothie, wash the peaches (it will take around 3), peel and remove the stone, then chop them into coarse pieces and set them aside.

The melon needs to be taken care of now. Cut it in half, take out the seeds, peel it, and chop it into pieces. Using a juicer, cut the lime in half and extract the juice. Gather the juice and set it away in a glass. Now put the peaches and melon in a blender. After adding the yogurt and lime juice, shut off and run the blender. Blend the mixture until it becomes creamy. It's time for your freshest yogurt smoothie!

12) Baked apples

Ingredients:
- Apples 4
- Brown sugar 40 g
- Honey 1 tbsp
- Ground cinnamon 1 tsp
- Sugar 1 tsp
- Lemons 1
- Water 50 g

Instructions

Cut the lemon into wedges and set aside before baking the apples.

Using a tiny knife, remove any remaining peel from the apples after removing the core and internal seeds. To prevent the peeled apples from becoming black, rub a lemon wedge over their surface. Transfer the brown sugar into a bowl and use the apples to coat the entire surface with the sugar. Arrange the apples in a well-sealed, ovenproof dish.

Dust the remaining brown sugar over the apple's exterior, being sure to get inside as well. Pour the water into the pan's bottom and spread the cinnamon over it to stop the sugar from burning and the apples from sticking. For thirty minutes, bake the apples at 200 °C in a static oven that has been warmed. Once the specified cooking time has elapsed, take out the pan and drizzle one tablespoon of honey over the apples' surface to enhance their shine.

Bake for an additional ten minutes at 200 °C. After baking, remove the pan of baked apples from the oven and dust with powdered sugar to enhance their

appearance. Drizzle the cooked apples with
the cooking juices and serve them hot.

CONCLUSION

Gastritis is used to describe a group of disorders with one feature in common, inflammation of the gastric mucosa. Today, in fact, in addition to being a discomfort that affects men and women of every race, age, and social rank, gastritis manifests itself in different forms: some gastritis sufferers complain of simple and temporary heartburn; in others, however, the disorder causes aerophagia, dyspepsia, loss of appetite, up to degenerate into severe and disabling symptoms such as diarrhea, abdominal cramps, meteorism, halitosis, and vomiting. The triggering cause intensely conditions the type of symptoms and the intensity with which they occur. Fortunately, in most cases, mild gastritis is quickly resolved with lifestyle correction. Other times, however, where the disease takes on a chronic or particularly aggressive connotation, the therapy must be more drastic. In both cases, especially if intense, the malaise felt must not be neglected but submitted to the attention of the doctor, both to avoid unnecessary suffering and because, even in a minority of people, the onset of heartburn, cramps, and Abdominal pain can be a sign of a more severe condition that can pose significant risks to overall health. It is advisable to change your lifestyle and diet, and this guide offers many useful tips on preventing gastritis with proper nutrition.